JOURNEY

JOURNEY

A SIMPLE ROADMAP FOR NEWLY
DIAGNOSED CANCER PATIENTS AND
THEIR FAMILIES

KATISHA VANCE, MD, FACP

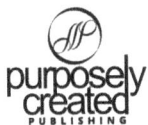

purposely
created
PUBLISHING

JOURNEY
Published by Purposely Created Publishing Group™
Copyright © 2020 Katisha Vance
All rights reserved.

Printed in the United States of America
ISBN: 978-1-64484-207-2

To my late grandmother, Mattie Lou Stinson (1922–1986), who taught me the importance of hard work, perseverance, and the art of making a lot from a little. Thank you to Al, Ryan, and Olivia for encouraging me to be brave and to take imperfect action.

Table of Contents

Foreword

You've just received the news. You turn to your family member, your doctor, and anyone in the room with a look of disbelief, anger, confusion, and sadness, all in an instant. They say that word, "cancer," and you imagine a bald head, dark eye bags, and an IV drip keeping you alive through the oncoming storm. It's not your fault this happened to you. But you're in for a shock: cancer can't rob you of everything. Most people who are battling cancer today have normal complexions and lifestyles, and may become just a tad more stubborn. ***You will become one of the strongest people you will ever encounter in your life.*** Your diagnosis isn't the end of the world; people walk past the hospital or clinic you are in, blissfully unaware that your life is coming to a halt. But make note of this: that halt is *temporary.* What you decide to do in your time here in the universe is *eternal.*

As a jovial eighteen year old who had only heard of cancer in textbooks, being slammed with a diagnosis made me defer a semester in college and cost me six months of anguish and sickness, but the people it made me encounter made that experience a little more bearable. I'm not here to tell you exactly how to deal with this new change. It's scary as hell, it's so uncertain, and you have no idea what to do. But if you do anything in this new journey, you need to surround yourself with good people. A support system will be the difference between life and death sometimes. You will learn so many medical terms, you might be eligible for medical school. You'll make lifelong friends in treatment rooms. You'll see kindness blossom from strangers from all walks of life, making your life easier. Cancer makes us look at life in a new lens that we've been forced to accept, but that doesn't mean you have to accept it lying down. I recommend staring it square in the eyes and fighting. Are you ready for it? If not, you'll learn how to be.

God bless,
Sarah Margaret Veres, Age Nineteen
Someone Who's Been There

Introduction

My maternal grandmother, Mattie Lou Stinson, was my first example of what it meant to be a strong, smart, and fearless woman. Though she only had an eighth grade education, my grandma Mattie could figure out anything. She and my sharecropping grandfather, Eddie, raised twelve children in Waugh, Alabama, on a meager income. Because my grandparents knew how to make a lot from a little, my mother, aunts, and uncles have few memories of going without the things they needed. At barely five feet tall, Mrs. Mattie, as she was affectionately called, could outwork the strongest man. For years, she worked as a domestic during the day and cared for her large family in the evenings.

My grandma Mattie was diagnosed with Stage 4 colon cancer in 1985, many months after complaining to doctors that she just did not feel like herself. They simply told her that she had "pains of life" and was "tired from having raised twelve kids." An exploratory surgery several months later told the real story: Grandma Mattie had metastatic colon cancer that was invading her liver, lungs, and entire abdominal cavity. My family and I were devastated by the shocking news of my grandmother's cancer diagnosis. We felt helpless and completely numb. We had no idea about what we needed to do. We did not know what to ask or who we should trust. Despite taking chemotherapy, my grandmother's cancer continued to grow wildly. She went on hospice in late July 1986.

On August 2, 1986, at the age of sixty-four, Mattie Lou Stinson died peacefully surrounded by family and friends.

Because of the helplessness that my family felt with my grandmother's terminal colon cancer diagnosis, I have sought to change the narrative for families facing a new cancer diagnosis. My mission is to teach patients and families how to navigate the cancer journey from diagnosis to treatment without fear and uncertainty. My purpose in being a cancer physician is to help someone else's Mattie.

CHAPTER 1

Understanding a Cancer Diagnosis: From a Patient's Perspective

Cancer. The word strikes fear in over seventeen million patients and their families worldwide every year. For some, that fear can be overwhelming to the point of inaction. "I am afraid!" becomes "I am giving up because surely there is no hope." However, in order to take the necessary steps to manage a cancer diagnosis, fear and anxiety must take a back seat to grit, determination, and perseverance. With the proper information and after dispelling some myths, it is possible to live well with and through a cancer diagnosis. I want to show you how!

Simply put, cancer is the uncontrolled growth of rogue cells in the body. That uncontrolled growth of abnormal cells can eventually harm normal cells or organs to the point that they no longer function properly. Human beings are so wonderfully designed that every cell in the body has a predetermined life span. New cells divide and grow to replace dead or dying cells all over the body. When this system is out of balance, because of genetic, environmental, or other complex influences, a cancer can develop. An invasive cancer or tumor not only grows at the location where it started, it also has the potential to spread to other vital organs. This local growth is problematic because it eventually causes the organ to not function properly. Likewise, when cancer spreads to other organs, it causes further organ dysfunction.

Consider this: A patient has a new diagnosis of lung cancer, meaning that the cancer started in the lungs. Though the cancer or tumor started in the lungs, it has the potential to spread to other organs like the liver, the brain, or the bones. When this happens, it is still lung cancer, but the terms *metastatic* or *Stage 4* are used to describe the lung cancer. The terms metastatic and Stage 4 are interchangeable.

TERMS THAT YOU MAY HEAR:

1. **Cancer:** Wild and uncontrolled growth of abnormal cells in the body.
2. **Chemotherapy:** Medicine or treatment that goes all over the body to treat cancer or to prevent the recurrence of cancer. Chemotherapy can be given by vein (intravenous or IV) or in a pill form (taken by mouth) depending on the type of cancer being treated.
3. **Clinical Trial:** Scientific studies used to find better, more effective treatments for diseases like cancer.
4. **Hematologist:** A doctor trained to diagnose and treat benign (noncancerous) and malignant (like leukemias and lymphomas) blood disorders or conditions.
5. **Medical oncologist:** A doctor trained to diagnose and treat cancer and the complications of cancer using chemotherapy, immunotherapy, hormone therapy, supportive care and other medications. Medical oncologists are also trained to assist with issues related to end-of-life care.
6. **Radiation oncologist:** A doctor trained to use radiation to treat cancer and complications of cancer. Radiation

TERMS THAT YOU MAY HEAR: (cont'd)

oncologists work closely with hematologists, surgical and medical oncologists to care for cancer patients.

7. **Radiation:** Local treatment using radiation for the treatment of a tumor/mass/cancer. Radiation treatment can be used in different settings: alone, after chemotherapy or in conjunction (at the same time) with chemotherapy.

8. **Stage:** Helps to describe how much of the body is affected by a cancer. It may consider the size of a tumor or mass, whether there are lymph nodes involved or whether the cancer has spread to other organs. In some cases, especially blood cancers like lymphoma or multiple myeloma, stage can also involve measuring specific blood tests.

9. **Surgical oncologist:** A doctor/surgeon trained in the diagnosis and treatment of cancer. A surgical oncologist may biopsy a tumor or mass for diagnosis or s/he may surgically remove the tumor or mass as a treatment.

10. **Tumor:** A mass of abnormal cells that can be cancerous (malignant) or benign (non-cancerous); sometimes the words mass, tumor and cancer are used interchangeably.

Why is stage important? There are several reasons why the stage of a cancer matters. First, the stage can help to determine if a cancer is curable. In very general terms, Stage 4 solid cancers or tumors, like breast, colon, lung, uterine, or ovarian cancer, are **usually** not curable. However, in patients who are otherwise well, therapy to slow the disease or to prevent symptoms (palliation) while prolonging life can and should be considered. So, when an oncologist (a doctor trained in cancer medicine) says that a cancer is **treatable** but not curable, they are suggesting that there are effective treatments available, like chemotherapy, to help shrink the cancer and perhaps slow the growth of cancer in other areas of the body for an unknown, but limited, amount of time.

Stage can also help to determine which therapies are appropriate. For some Stage 1 cancers, like colorectal cancer, surgery alone may be curative; however, that may not be the case for other types, such as a high-risk Stage 1 breast cancer, which may require a combination of chemotherapy and/or radiation after surgery. Depending on the stage of a cancer, a medical oncologist or hematologist may recommend chemotherapy. Additionally, a radiation oncologist may recommend radiation therapy.

Chemotherapy is a **systemic medicine or treatment** that goes throughout the body to fight cancer cells. These drugs are commonly delivered intravenously through specialized central intravenous catheters (IVs) called mediports that are placed just under the skin. Chemotherapy can also be given by a regular IV that is put in place in the office. Some chemotherapy agents can even be given by mouth. When a cancer is metastatic, meaning that it has spread to other vital organs outside of where it started, chemotherapy is often recommended. Chemotherapy can also be recommended in the curative setting when a cancer has been completely removed surgically but there is an unacceptably high risk of recurrence. An example of this is stage 3 colorectal cancer. When chemotherapy is given after surgery, the goal is to lower the risk of cancer recurrence.

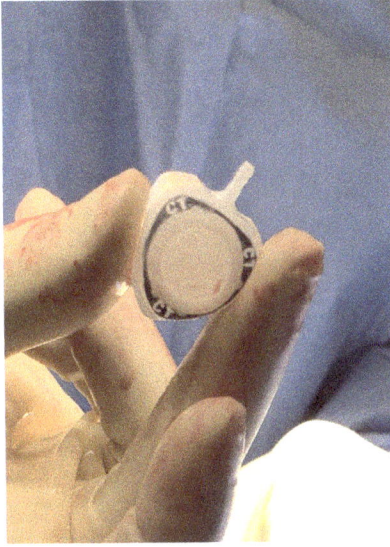

a) A mediport (portacath) is placed in a small pocket underneath the skin; this portacath is connected to a catheter in a central vein

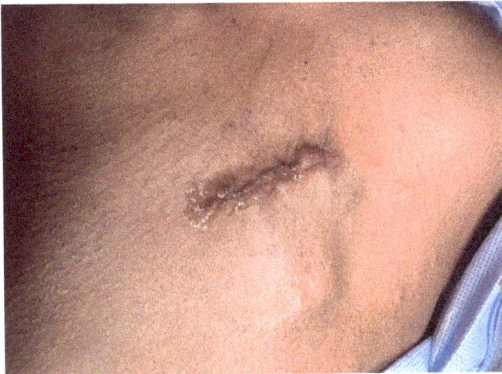

b) Chest wall showing an unaccessed mediport

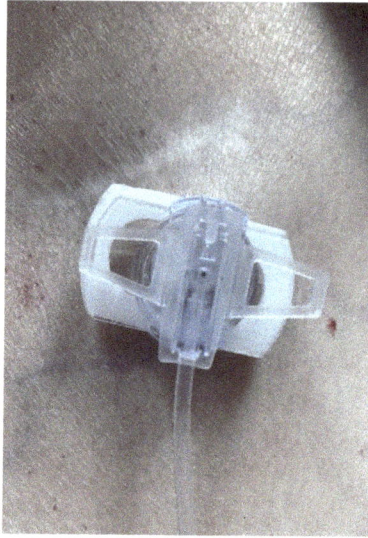

c) Chest wall showing a mediport accessed with a Huber needle

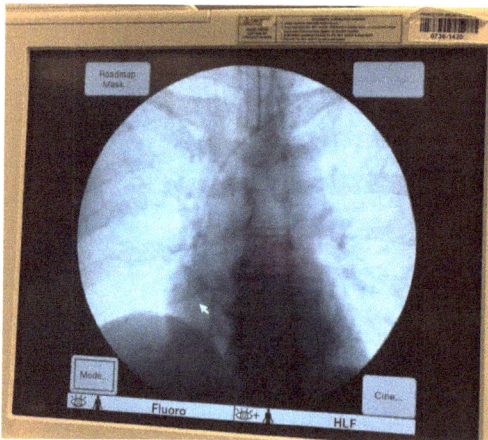

d) The tip of the mediport catheter (arrow) is in the region of the superior vena cava

> **THE ROAD TO CHEMOTHERAPY:**
>
> 1. After surgery (adjuvant) to lower the risk of cancer recurrence
>
> 2. Before surgery (neoadjuvant) to shrink the size of a cancer prior to the surgery being performed
>
> 3. In cases of metastatic cancer (examples include breast, colon, lung, uterine) to shrink cancer, to reduce or prevent symptoms, or to prolong life
>
> 4. In blood cancers like lymphoma or leukemia with the intent to cure or to prolong life and reduce symptoms

Chemotherapy is most beneficial to patients who are highly functional with a good performance status. The performance status is a measure of a cancer patient's overall wellbeing and level of function. It helps to determine if a patient should consider taking chemotherapy, or if chemotherapy is more likely to cause harm. There are two scales used to measure a patient's functional or performance status: the Karnofsky Performance Status Scale (KPS) and the Eastern Cooperative Oncology Group (ECOG) performance status scale. Your doctor may use either.

The KPS uses a scale between 0–100 percent. A low KPS is associated with a poorer prognosis and lower chance of survival. A KPS of 60–100 percent is desirable for patients who are considering chemotherapy.

KPS (%)	Functional status
100	Normal, no complaints.
90	Normal activity, minor signs/symptoms of disease.
80	Normal activity with effort.
70	Able to perform self-care, but unable to work or carry out activities.
60	Able to perform majority of self-care with occasional help.
50	Unable to perform most self-care; requires frequent medical care.
40	Disabled; requires special assistance.
30	Severely disabled; hospitalization indicated.
20	Critically ill; hospitalization necessary with active supportive treatment.
10	Approaching death.
0	Dead.

The ECOG scale ranges from 0 to 5. An ECOG performance status of 0, 1, or 2 is desirable for patients who are considering chemotherapy. Studies have shown that these are the patients most likely to benefit from aggressive treatment. Many clinical trials also require that patients have a good performance status, usually ECOG 0, 1, or 2, to participate. We will talk about clinical trials in Chapter 7.

ECOG Performance Status	Functional Status
0	Fully active, able to carry on all pre-disease performance without restriction.
1	Restricted in physically strenuous activity, but walking and able to do light or seated work in the home or office.
2	Walking and capable of all self-care but unable to work. Up and out of bed or a chair for more than 50% of waking hours.
3	Capable of only limited self-care; confined to bed or chair more than 50% of waking hours.
4	Completely disabled. Unable to carry on any self-care. Totally confined to bed or chair.
5	Dead.

Neoadjuvant chemotherapy is chemotherapy that is given before surgery. There are specific situations with breast, rectal, and other gastrointestinal cancers where the surgeon and radiation oncologist may refer patients for chemotherapy before surgery. An example of when neoadjuvant chemotherapy may be useful is in some cases of breast cancer. Neoadjuvant chemotherapy can be given to shrink the size of the cancer if a patient desires less surgery, like a lumpectomy/partial mastectomy. Also, if the surgeon is concerned that complete removal of a tumor or cancer is impossible without leaving cancer behind, then neoadjuvant chemotherapy may be desirable. Remember, every case is different.

Because cancer is so common and the treatments are often portrayed as being harsh or toxic, there is a lot of interest in a "natural approach" to cancer care. Natural treatment can mean different things, so make sure that you are clear with your doctor about alternative therapies that you are using or considering. Natural therapies to help with side effects of cancer or cancer treatment can be tricky. For example, many women with bothersome hot flashes, vaginal dryness, or mood swings from breast cancer treatment (tamoxifen, letrozole, anastrozole, exemestane, or faslodex, for example) will try natural products to help with symptoms. The problem is that these natural products are either estrogen-based products or estrogen mimickers that can work against the cancer treatment. More worrisome are the centers that offer "the cancer cure," using unproven, unscientific methods of detoxifying or cleansing the body of cancer. Centers like these prey on the vulnerability of the cancer patient and should be avoided.

Radiation therapy is **local treatment** that can be used in combination with chemotherapy or alone. Radiation can be given for curative treatment or to alleviate symptoms like pain. The medical and radiation oncologists will frequently work together to figure out the best treatment strategy. Other medical professionals that contribute to the diagnosis and treatment of cancer are general surgeons and surgical oncologists, pathologists, and radiologists.

THE FIRST VISIT

Here are a few tips for your first visit, along with questions that you should ask or expect on your initial encounter with the medical or radiation oncologist:

1. First, do not come alone if possible. Bring a supportive family member or friend to help process the information that you will be receiving. Too many family or friends can be disruptive, however, so limit the number of people who come with you to two or three. Avoid bringing small children, if possible. Turn off cellphones or other disruptive devices.

2. If you are interested in recording the visit, ask permission from your doctor first.

3. Expect for the first visit to be longer than usual. If your visit will affect a mealtime or a typical medication time, plan for that accordingly. Likewise, if your visit will include a chemotherapy treatment, anticipate a long day (in some cases four to five hours).

4. Avoid the temptation to seek medical advice from Dr. Google, chat rooms, or social media. Family members and friends who are well-meaning may be tempted to give you advice as well. My advice is to be knowledgeable

about your disease with the help of your medical oncologist or radiation oncologist. They can refer you to reputable sources if you feel that you need additional explanations about your disease or treatment.

5. The relationship that you form with your physician is an important one that should be grounded in trust and mutual respect.

This is a good time to address second opinions. Very often, patients and their families are interested in hearing from other medical providers to make sure that they are getting the best treatment advice. My recommendation on this topic is very simple: because cancer is so complex, it is not unreasonable to get a second opinion before starting your treatment. Second opinions may allow for consideration of a clinical trial (discussed later in the book) with new therapies. In general, however, FDA-approved therapies for all cancer types will follow specific and well-accepted national guidelines. Whatever the case, be sure that getting another opinion will not lead to significant time delays in initiating treatment. Sometimes getting a second opinion can be done very quickly with a telemedicine or virtual medicine consultation. An internet search for reputable cancer-trained physicians who provide second opinions can also be done quickly and easily. A word to the wise, however—do not get distracted by charlatans and quacks offering the "cancer cure" for a significant fee.

6. Have a good grasp of your personal medical history and your family's medical history. The most important family members to have detailed history on are your parents, siblings, and, if possible, both sets of grandparents. Know if your parents, siblings, or grandparents had a cancer diagnosis, what type it was, and their age at diagnosis, if possible.

7. Prepare a detailed list of the medications that you currently take and keep it in your wallet, purse, or smartphone for easy reference. This should include herbal and over-the-counter medications. Know the name, dose, and frequency of administration of each medication. This is important to avoid potentially severe drug interactions.

8. Know your drug and food allergies. What happens if you are exposed to the drug or food?

9. A list of important things to know about your cancer:

   - Type of cancer
     * Important markers, genetic mutations
     * Is genetic testing indicated?
   - Stage
   - Treatment recommendations
     * Drugs (IV and oral)
     * How often?

- * Is radiation indicated?

- * Important side effects

- * Side effects that are considered emergent or urgent

- Treating for **cure or palliation** (slowing incurable disease, preventing symptoms, extending life)

- If not treating for cure, discuss benefits of a living will (see example in appendix)

- Should family members be tested for this cancer?

- Should family members have genetic screening?

10. Ask about surveillance strategies. How will you know if the treatment is or is not working? Will there be scans once chemotherapy has completed? Why or why not?

11. Are there support groups available?

12. Is there a financial counselor to help manage the economic impact of your cancer diagnosis?

13. Acknowledge habits that may affect treatment effectiveness, like smoking, alcohol use/abuse, or drug dependence. Ask for help with quitting, if needed.

14. Does your doctor participate in clinical trials? Is it appropriate to consider a trial in this setting?

15. For women/men of childbearing age, what are the implications of treatment on future fertility?

CHAPTER 2

Cancer Is Emotionally Distressing

It will come as no surprise that a cancer diagnosis is emotionally and psychologically distressing. Sometimes patients, physicians, and family members are so focused on the physical aspects of the cancer, and how the cancer is responding to chemotherapy, that the emotional toll of cancer is greatly underestimated or not recognized at all. This was never more apparent to me than in 2017, when one of my patients committed suicide. Luke* (name changed for anonymity) ended his life with a self-inflicted gunshot wound at a time when his cancer was responding to treatment with minimal side effects from therapy. The last phone call that I had with his wife was to say that his cancer was shrinking on the CAT scans. As I reflected, however, I realized that Luke had been struggling to keep up with the demands of his job, and, more importantly, he was dealing with alcoholism. Despite a referral to psychiatry for evaluation, and their best efforts, Luke committed suicide. My patient's death by suicide made me recognize how little time and emphasis is spent on discussing the emotional distress associated with a cancer diagnosis. With over seventeen million cancer survivors worldwide as of January 2019, and a projection of over twenty-seven million cancer diagnoses by 2040, an emphasis on the emotional impact of cancer must become a priority. (https://cancercontrol.cancer.gov/ocs/statistics/index.html)

A cancer diagnosis often comes with feelings of hopelessness and loss of control. Patients and family members readily acknowledge that they are often at a complete loss for words, and feel even more uncertain about the course of action that they should take, when a cancer diagnosis is made. Here are a few tips for patients, friends, and family members:

1. Acknowledge that you don't know exactly what to say. Allow the patient to express his/her feelings instead.

2. "I know exactly how you feel" may seem like the empathetic thing to say. The truth, however, is that every patient's cancer journey is different. Even if you have previous experience with a cancer diagnosis, allow the patient to create their own.

3. Avoid stories of patients with the same or a similar cancer diagnosis. Hearing about a good outcome can create false hope or unrealistic expectations. Likewise, stories of a bad outcome can cause unnecessary worry and rob a patient of hope. The bottom line: everyone must write his or her own story.

4. Because everyone has an opinion about a cancer diagnosis, be cautious about the information that you receive. Well-meaning family and friends can unintentionally cause anxiety and confusion with treatment recommendations and stories of other cancer patients.

5. Seek out a support group. Many patients will initially frown upon joining a support group, saying something like "I don't want to sit and talk to strangers about cancer all day." However, talking and interacting with others who are going through or who have gone through similar journeys can be very helpful. Some of the best and most meaningful interactions that I have witnessed happened very organically amongst patients in the infusion room. What did they all have in common? They were all walking through a journey with cancer.

6. Consider engaging a therapist or psychiatrist. Sometimes it is helpful to be able to express one's fears, anxieties, and regrets to an impartial listener. A therapist or psychiatrist who is trained to help patients with chronic or incurable illnesses can be invaluable.

7. Consider counseling from a minister or other spiritual advisor. As a Christian in the Deep South, prayer and spirituality are a very real part of my life and the lives of my family and friends. It is important to recognize that a cancer diagnosis can push some toward spirituality, while for others, who see cancer as some form of punishment, it can cause them to turn away from God. A minister or spiritual counselor can help sort out these conflicting feelings.

8. Be honest and open with your physician. Doctors are trained to look for signs and symptoms of depression.

Feelings of sadness, failure to enjoy one's usual hobbies, excessive sleeping or lack of sleeping, and changes in weight and appetite can all be signs or symptoms of depression. However, these findings can be subtle or easily explained away by a cancer diagnosis or by the side effects of the treatment of cancer. That is why talking about these signs or symptoms in detail with your doctor is important.

9. Know that antidepressants can be helpful. For so many patients, the stigma associated with depression and mental illness keeps them from asking for the help that they need. An antidepressant or antianxiety medication may be the answer to get you through the lowest points of a cancer diagnosis.

10. Tell your doctor right away if you are considering suicide or if you have a plan to end your life. Help is available! The National Suicide Hotline is available twenty-four hours a day, every day, at 1-800-273-8255.

THE TOUGH QUESTIONS

There are a lot of tough questions that nobody asks when there is a new cancer diagnosis. I have discovered over the years that patients and family want to ask things like "How long, doctor?"; "What if we do nothing, doctor?"; or "What would you do if you were in our shoes?" But usually, they don't. They don't ask the tough questions because often the answers are hard. They don't ask the tough questions because the answers make the whole scenario much more real and in your face. I have long thought that the tough questions come out slowly, almost in a trickle, because that is all that we as humans can handle. This approach of trickling out information is not deliberate, but it is often criticized, especially by non-cancer physicians. Here's how it usually goes: A physician delivers the news that cancer has been discovered. The treatment options are discussed. If the cancer is incurable, there is the transition into the ways that the cancer can be treated or managed, as well as the response rates to treatment. Inevitably, a family member or the patient, trying to bring lightness to a dark conversation, will offer a ray of hope. Usually it's a comment like, "But you're strong. You can beat this." Then it happens. We all proceed without asking those tough questions. At least for a while.

Elizabeth* was one of the first patients that I cared for out of fellowship training. She was a proud octogenarian who was a leader in her community and her church. Elizabeth was referred to me by a physician who I respected tremendously as a long-time servant in an underserved local community and hospital. The orders were clear when he referred Elizabeth: "Take good care of her. I am counting on you." Elizabeth had Stage 4 diffuse large B-cell lymphoma. I still remember how calm she was when she got the diagnosis. That calm never wavered, even as we discussed how difficult her treatment would be. She endured a bone marrow biopsy and chemotherapy without ever complaining. Like so many patients who I have treated since then, Elizabeth never asked the hard questions—at least not at first. After the first four cycles of treatment, Elizabeth had a partial response, but it came at a cost. She was quite weakened by the treatment, and because of her frailty, she was not able to go on with any additional treatment. On my last visit with her, she finally asked, "Doctor, how long do I have?" I estimated that because of her weakened overall condition from not eating or drinking, Elizabeth would likely only have a few weeks to live. I told her this with a great deal of reluctance, but she accepted my answer with the grace that I had grown to expect from her. My reluctance came out of the fear that Elizabeth would give up, and I believe that is what she did. She died a few short weeks after our conversation.

In the case of another very memorable patient, Thomas*, the tough questions came early in the course of his diagnosis. Thomas was in his fifties with Stage 4 lung cancer. His presentation was very unusual, in that his lung cancer had spread to his colon. As I was visiting with him in the intensive care unit early one morning, he asked me, "Doc, how long do you think I have to live?" I hesitated momentarily, considering the entire picture. Thomas was young, but his disease was very aggressive. I said to him, "I think that you only have a few months to live, maybe three or four at best." He looked at me with wide eyes and said, "Damn, doc. Why did you have to be so honest?"

Dealing with the tough questions presents quite a dilemma for the patient, family members, and doctors. There is a fine balance of not wanting to mislead or relay false expectations, but also having the desire to give hope. Amos Bailey, MD, who was my palliative care attending at the Veteran's Administration Hospital in Birmingham, Alabama, introduced me to this Benjamin Disraeli quote: "I am prepared for the worst, but hope for the best." That is what I want for all my patients, and for anyone reading this book. Here are a few tips:

1. Don't be afraid to ask the tough questions. If your doctor has said that your cancer is incurable, it is okay to ask "How long do you think I have to live?"

2. Understand that our answers are educated guesses, based on experience with other patients in similar situations. Because no two patients are alike, our "guesses" are flawed at best.

3. A cancer diagnosis, even stage 4, does not have to be an immediate death sentence. However, use it as an opportunity to plan. Do you have a trust or will? Have you completed a living will? Take the time to speak with a qualified attorney who may be able to handle your estate planning at a reasonable cost.

4. Evaluate your perspective on life. Many patients with a diagnosis of incurable cancer stop focusing on the small stuff. Faith, family, and friends may take on an entirely new level of importance.

CHAPTER 3
Side Effects of Treatment

There are times when the fear of the side effects of treatment outweighs the fear of cancer itself. I have seen patients decline potentially life-extending or even cancer-curing treatment because of misleading or inaccurate information about chemotherapy or radiation therapy. I start every discussion about chemotherapy with some simple facts: There is no such thing as a drug that does not have potential side effects. However, because of better supportive care medications and targeted therapies, chemotherapy is increasingly more effective and well-tolerated.

There are many side effects that can be associated with chemotherapeutic drugs. Some side effects, like fatigue, are expected but are manageable. I will address fatigue as a chronic side effect later in Chapter 9. Other side effects, like neutropenia (low white blood cell count), nausea, vomiting, alopecia (hair loss), neuropathy (nerve damage that causes numbness and tingling in the fingers or toes), and diarrhea, have effective management strategies that will be discussed here.

NEUTROPENIA

Neutropenia, or a decrease in the white blood cell count, is an expected side effect of some chemotherapy treatments. With many regimens, a low white blood cell count occurs five to seven days after chemotherapy is given. In order to shorten the number of days that the white blood cell count is low, white blood cell growth factors can be given. White blood cell growth factors like Neupogen or Neulasta, when given in the appropriate setting, can help lower the risk of life-threatening infections. White blood cell growth factors do this by shortening the amount of time that the white blood cell count is low. It does not prevent the white blood cell count from dropping, however.

Because a low white blood cell count can increase the risk of infection, patients on chemotherapy should notify their doctor immediately for a temperature of 100.5 degrees Fahrenheit or greater, chills, or night sweats. These may be symptoms of an underlying infection, which can be life-threatening.

In addition to increasing the risk for infection, having neutropenia increases the risk for mucositis, or mouth sores. Generally, once the white blood cell count recovers, the mouth sores will resolve spontaneously. For symptom management of the mouth sores, it is recommended to avoid spicy or highly acidic foods or drinks. Additionally, some patients will find relief with analgesics like lidocaine found in Magic mouthwash, which is available by prescription. If mucositis is extremely severe, a patient may require hospitalization for maintenance of proper fluid status to prevent dehydration.

NAUSEA AND VOMITING

Whenever chemotherapy patients are portrayed on television or in the movies, they are usually seen or heard throwing up. With the availability of newer and better anti-nausea medications, nausea and vomiting are unacceptable side effects. Something to remember is that nausea and vomiting are two different symptoms that arise from different areas of the brain. Nausea is the uncomfortable feeling that we get in the pit of our stomach that usually signals that vomiting is about to happen. Both symptoms are miserable.

The best treatment for nausea and vomiting is prevention. Before you are given chemotherapy, ask your doctor what anti-nausea medications you will receive. For certain drugs, the risk of nausea and vomiting is extremely high. Chemotherapy drugs like cisplatin and Adriamycin, for example, are much more likely to cause nausea and vomiting than 5-fluorouracil and paclitaxel. Because of that, stronger, longer-lasting anti-nausea drugs with different mechanisms of action are more likely to be given before administration of cisplatin and Adriamycin.

It is also important to recognize that some patients are more likely to have nausea and vomiting with chemotherapy than others. For those who may be prone to motion sickness or for women who had difficulty with extreme nausea and vomiting during pregnancy, your doctor may provide additional options to prevent nausea and vomiting.

Once nausea and vomiting occur, several things are important to remember: 1) Avoid foods or smells that may trigger ongoing symptoms, 2) Consider using an anti-nausea suppository (given per rectum) or a tablet that dissolves in the mouth instead of one that you may vomit up before it starts to work, and 3) Drink plenty of water and electrolyte replacement drinks to avoid dehydration.

Nausea and vomiting from chemotherapy are most likely to occur in the first four days after treatment. As such, scheduled anti-nausea medicine for the first four days after treatment is helpful. Remember, prevention is the key! If nausea and vomiting occur more than a week after chemotherapy, discuss it with your doctor, as other causes of nausea and vomiting should be considered.

DIARRHEA

Another common gastrointestinal (GI) side effect is diarrhea. Chemotherapy drugs like 5-fluorouracil and irinotecan are commonly associated with diarrhea. Treatment with over-the-counter (OTC) antidiarrheals like Imodium, Pepto-Bismol, or Kaopectate may helpful to stop diarrhea and prevent dehydration. If OTCs are not helpful, talk to your doctor about prescription antidiarrheal medications like Lomotil. Just like with nausea and vomiting, it is important to drink plenty of water or fluids with electrolytes to avoid dehydration.

Symptoms of dehydration include extreme thirst, not urinating often, dark or tea-colored urine, muscle cramps, dizziness

PUT A STOP TO NAUSEA AND VOMITING BEFORE IT STARTS:

1. Avoid sugary sweet, greasy/oily, or spicy foods.

2. Eat small meals, and eat more frequently. Try four to six small plate servings each day.

3. Avoid foods with strong odors. Being in another area while food is being prepared may help.

4. Take your time eating.

5. Avoid tightfitting clothes or undergarments.

6. Try peppermint or ginger candy to combat nausea.

7. A small meal before chemotherapy may be helpful.

8. Avoid lying down for two to three hours after eating.

9. Take your nausea medicine on time and as prescribed by your doctor.

10. Be sure to let your doctor know if you are struggling with nausea and vomiting!

or lightheadedness, especially when changing positions (from laying down to sitting up or sitting to standing).

If you have more than three or four loose bowel movements daily or if your stools are bloody, it is extremely important to report this to your doctor, as it may indicate a more serious problem. Let your doctor know if there has been recent antibiotic use before the onset of bloody diarrhea as well.

WHEN DIARRHEA HAS YOU ON THE RUN:

1. Drink a maintenance amount of water, Pedialyte, or diluted sports drink (one cup sports drink like Gatorade to one cup water)—see chart "How Much Water" on page 43—plus an additional six to eight ounces of liquid after each loose bowel movement.

2. Avoid sugary drinks or juices, coffee, and dairy products (including supplements like Boost or Ensure).

3. Eat high protein foods, such as lean meats (chicken, fish, turkey, beef), eggs, and potatoes.

4. Avoid high fiber foods, such as whole wheat products, cauliflower, green beans, root vegetables like carrots, dried beans, and peas.

5. Eat low fiber foods instead, such as white rice, white bread/toast, crackers, plain white pasta, fish, eggs, bananas, or other fruits without skins or seeds.

6. After a loose (unformed) or watery bowel movement, take Imodium, Kaopectate, or Pepto-Bismol. Diarrhea that does not respond to these agents may require a prescription antidiarrheal like Lomotil.

7. Call your doctor if the diarrhea is not responding to treatment measures, or if your heart is racing, your blood pressure is low, your urine output is down or appears dark, or if you are dizzy/lightheaded. These may be symptoms of dehydration.

NEUROPATHY

Neuropathy is a very troubling side effect that can be seen with multiple chemotherapy drug classes like taxanes (paclitaxel, docetaxel) and platinums (cisplatin, carboplatin, and oxaliplatin), just to name a few. The key with neuropathy is to have frequent discussions with your doctor about what you are experiencing. If you are having trouble buttoning your clothes, picking up small items, or turning pages in a book, your medication dose may need to be adjusted. For some patients, neuropathy can become so severe that they have difficulty walking or they experience frequent falls. Neuropathy can also become painful, leading to difficulties with sleep. When neuropathy becomes moderate or severe, you may get some relief with medications prescribed by your doctor. Remember, though, there is no such thing as a drug that does not have side effects! The drugs to treat neuropathy may have side effects that some patients find more intolerable than the neuropathy.

Other strategies that may help include wearing gloves in cold weather, using topical compounding ointments, and taking a complex of B vitamins. For patients being treated with oxaliplatin for colorectal or pancreatic cancer, the neuropathy is quite unique, as it is worse with exposure to cold. Patients on oxaliplatin are instructed to avoid touching, eating, or drinking anything colder than room temperature for five to seven days after each treatment. While the "shocking" feeling in the hands and throat is uncomfortable if something cold is touched or ingested, it is not typically life threatening. Wearing gloves to protect your hands and a scarf over your face and mouth can help to prevent discomfort, numbness, and tingling from cold air on cool days. In the most severe cases, neuropathy is a side effect that lingers for months and sometimes years as the nerves repair and regrow from chemotherapy damage. I advise patients to measure their progress in months, rather than in days or weeks.

SKIN CHANGES

Darkening of the skin of the face, the palms of the hands, and the soles of the feet is common with chemotherapy. These skin changes will frequently be seen along with nail changes, where there is a band extending from the base of the nail to the tip. These nail and skin changes can be seen in all patients; however, the changes may be more pronounced in patients of color. These changes are temporary and will go away with time when chemotherapy treatment has completed.

Lightening of the skin and hair has also been seen with certain chemotherapy drugs like tyrosine kinase inhibitors (Sunitinib is an example). As with other changes, these skin changes are temporary and go away when the chemotherapy treatment has completed.

Newer chemotherapeutic agents are known to cause dramatic skin changes. Cetuximab, used for colorectal and head and neck cancer, causes an often-severe rash that looks like acne. Interestingly, the development of the rash is associated with a good response to treatment.

Hand and foot syndrome can be seen with drugs like Xeloda and Doxil. With both drugs, the palms of the hands and the soles of the feet can become quite tender, red, and painful, with cracking and darkening of the skin. The best management for hand and foot syndrome is to use heavy lotions or emollients. The syndrome will go away with the discontinuation of Xeloda and Doxil.

With any chemotherapy drug, patients should be aware of increased skin sensitivity and increased risk for sunburn. I encourage a minimum sun protection factor (SPF) of 30 used at least thirty minutes prior to sun exposure. Additionally, wide-brimmed hats and limited to no sun exposure during the hottest parts of the day is recommended.

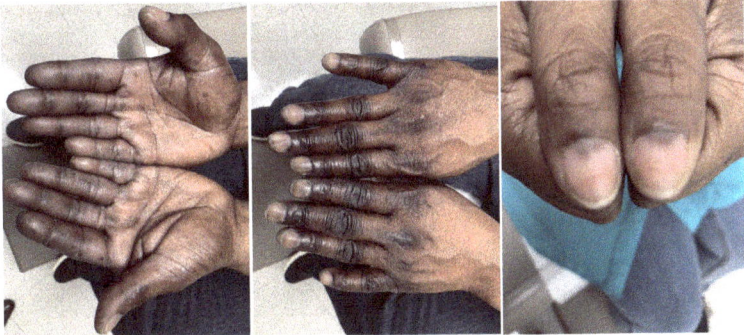

a, b) Chemotherapy skin changes, with darkening of the skin of the palms and tops of the hands. Similar changes are seen on the soles of the feet. These changes are not permanent, and the skin returns to normal when chemotherapy is discontinued.

c) Chemotherapy nail changes, with a dark band at the base of the nail. The dark band will continue to move out to the tip of the nails of the hands and feet.

HAIR LOSS/ALOPECIA

One of the more distressing side effects of chemotherapy drugs is hair loss, or alopecia. While not every drug or regimen causes hair loss, when it does occur, it is usually reversible. In some cases, the scalp can be very tender and painful when hair loss begins. The solution is quite simple—shave the remaining hair. Care should be taken to protect the scalp from excessive amounts of sun and harsh chemicals.

Loss of the eyelashes can also be expected with certain chemotherapy drugs. With the loss of eyelashes, be sure to wear sunglasses (or corrective lenses, if necessary) to protect your eyes from the dust, sand, or other fine particles in the air. Most patients will notice regrowth of hair after chemotherapy has completed.

NOW I'VE LOST IT!

1. Don't hesitate to shave your head once your hair begins to fall out. It may eliminate scalp irritation and tenderness.

2. Hair loss may begin just a few days after your first treatment.

3. Treat your scalp with care. Moisturize with lotions like Lubriderm or Eucerin. Use sunblock (at least SPF 30), hats, or scarves to protect from sunburn.

4. Ask your doctor for a prescription for a "hair prosthetic" or wig. They are covered by some insurance companies.

5. Know that it is normal—not vain—to be upset by hair loss. Nobody should tell you to "just get over it!"

DENTAL HEALTH

Chemotherapy, radiation, and supportive care medications can cause major problems with the teeth, gums, and jawbones. The body's ability to make saliva or spit may also be affected by both chemotherapy and radiation. Because saliva or spit has natural bacteria to protect the teeth and gums, when spit production goes down, patients may notice mouth sores, gum swelling, or inflammation. In addition, the teeth may become more susceptible to breakage, loosening, and cavities or decay.

Osteonecrosis of the jaw, or ONJ, is another serious problem seen with certain medicines used in cancer patients to prevent bone fractures or breaks. With ONJ, there is an exposed area of the jawbone that is no longer covered by the gums, usually occurring in an area where a tooth has been pulled or where other major dental work has been performed. ONJ can be painful, and it can be associated

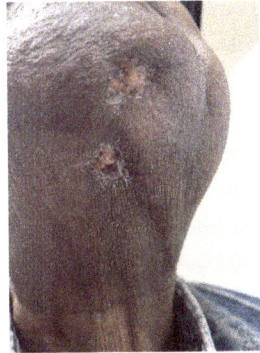

a) Osteonecrosis of the jaw (ONJ) after exposure to denosumab (Xgeva).

with constant drainage requiring use of antibiotics. ONJ is associated with medications like bisphosphonates (zoledronic acid, pamidronate, alendronate, risedronate, ibandronate) or denosumab (Prolia, Xgeva). Once beginning a bisphosphonate or denosumab, major dental work like tooth extractions

35

(getting a tooth pulled), root canals, crowns, bridges, etc., will need to be put on hold for several months if possible. Routine cleanings and treatments to prevent cavities, however, are acceptable and encouraged. Let your dentist know if you are taking any of these medications.

JUST SMILE!

1. If possible, see your dentist before starting chemotherapy or radiation for a prophylactic cleaning or other necessary dental work.
2. Consult with your dentist about fluoride treatments.
3. Drink water from the tap. It has fluoride!
4. Cut back on or eliminate concentrated sugars and sweets.
5. Brush and floss at least twice daily, after each meal if possible.
6. Let your dentist know if you are taking a bisphosphonate or denosumab at each visit.
7. Avoid biting or chewing hard or sticky substances like hard candies or ice that may break a tooth.
8. Clean your teeth and under dentures or partials with a soft (not hard) toothbrush.
9. Brush your tongue. This will help with unusual tastes or dark discoloration of the tongue.
10. Avoid mouthwashes that contain alcohol. They can cause a lot of pain and discomfort when mouth sores are present.
11. Magic Mouthwash or other medicated rinses can help with pain from mouth sores and thrush.

EXTREMITY SWELLING

Swelling of the extremities, especially the legs, is commonly seen in cancer patients. Sometimes the swelling is due to non-cancer related causes, like IV fluids given in the hospital or office, medications to treat other conditions, or a low protein state. It is important, however, to rule out a potentially life-threatening blood clot or deep venous thrombosis (DVT) as the cause of extremity swelling in patients with active cancer or who are on chemotherapy. Drugs like Tamoxifen can increase the risk of a DVT, though this is a rare side effect. Additionally, placement of intravenous (IV) devices like mediports or peripherally inserted central catheters (PICC lines) can increase the risk of a DVT.

A DVT must be ruled out if there is tenderness, redness, or swelling in an arm or leg. A DVT is diagnosed with ultrasound and treated with blood thinning medications. For cancer patients, DVTs are sometimes managed differently than in the general population.

CHAPTER 4

Eating and Hydrating with Cancer

There has been a great deal written and discussed about how cancer patients should eat. Many patients start out with lists of things that they have been warned to avoid—ranging from anything with sugar to meats in general. Once chemotherapy starts, however, it can be difficult to keep all these restrictions in place. The foods that were commonly eaten and enjoyed before a cancer diagnosis may not taste the same, and the smells from others may be nauseating. I suggest keeping things as simple as possible.

First, the goal is to maintain your weight. This is not the season for dramatic weight loss (if it can be avoided) or weight gain (it happens more than you would guess!).

Next, eat plenty of protein! I would recommend 0.8–1 mg/kg of protein (milligrams of protein per kilogram you weigh) daily while on chemotherapy. Plant-based protein from sources like beans, peas, nuts, and seeds is best. However, protein from lean meats like chicken, turkey, and fish is also helpful. Beef and pork can be eaten sparingly or not at all, if that is your preference.

To prevent nausea and vomiting, avoid preparing or eating overly sweet or spicy foods or meals with strong odors. If possible, stay out of the area where food is being prepared to avoid offensive smells that might trigger nausea or vomiting.

> **HOW MUCH PROTEIN?**
>
> Consider a patient who weighs 150 pounds:
>
> To get weight in kilograms: 150÷2.2 = 68 kg
>
> Amount of protein per day: 68 kg×0.8 or 1 = Between 54 and 68 grams of protein per day

Next, consider doing the bulk of your shopping in the perimeter aisles of the grocery store. This is where you will find whole, natural foods like fresh fruits and vegetables, meats, and dairy products. Whole foods are foods made up of only one ingredient. With a cancer diagnosis, properly washed fresh fruits and vegetables, as opposed to processed foods, are preferable.

When preparing foods, consider using fresh herbs like rosemary, sage, basil, or oregano for seasoning. Lemon or lime juice added to fish or chicken can help make a meal more appetizing, especially if food has a bitter or metallic taste. Avoid acidic juices like orange juice, spicy condiments like hot sauce, or excessive amounts of pepper that can make mouth sores or mucositis from chemotherapy feel much worse.

Another tip is to use plastic utensils, as opposed to metal forks and spoons, to avoid the metallic, bitter taste that some patients experience.

Avoid spending tons of money on the "cancer cure" diet. There are lots of unscrupulous people anxious to capitalize on patients with a cancer diagnosis. Eating well with cancer should be based on simple, common-sense principles. If it has one ingredient, it is a whole food and reasonable to eat. Good examples of whole foods are fresh fruits and vegetables. If a food or food product has ingredients that you cannot pronounce or have never heard of, it is likely a processed food. Avoid or eat very limited amounts of processed foods.

The day of chemotherapy: It is fine and even recommended to eat on the morning or day of your chemotherapy treatment. This may lower your risk of chemotherapy-associated nausea and vomiting. If you plan to eat in the infusion or treatment area, take foods that do not have a strong odor so as not to offend other patients.

BREAKFAST IS A GO!

1. Oatmeal with fresh fruit and/or nuts (fiber and protein)
2. Grits and eggs (vitamins A, C, protein, folate)
3. Steak and eggs (protein, folate, iron)

After chemotherapy: Difficulties with food may not happen for two or three days after chemotherapy. The most common problems that patients encounter after chemotherapy are related to nausea, vomiting, decreased appetite, and altered taste sensation.

As discussed earlier, there are a few simple things you can try to prevent nausea and vomiting. Avoid foods that have a strong odor, or are very greasy or spicy. Try not to skip meals. If you are not able to eat a regular meal, consider a fruit- or vegetable-based smoothie instead. Avoid dairy or milk-based products if you are lactose intolerant. Sometimes large meals are overwhelming; try eating more frequent, small, saucer-sized meals instead.

Don't stress out over food. If the first few days after chemotherapy are a struggle, know that your appetite will get better. Staying adequately hydrated (see page 43) on those days when you are not eating very much is extremely important. If you are having diarrhea or vomiting, staying properly hydrated can be even more challenging. If so, in addition to the usual fluid intake, add six to eight ounces of water or Pedialyte after each loose bowel movement to maintain hydration. If you are experiencing vomiting, go slowly with your fluid intake.

Caffeinated drinks like coffee, tea, or soft drinks can worsen fluid loss. Furthermore, the gas bubbles in carbonated drinks can make nausea and vomiting worse. With that in mind, consider water, fruit or vegetable juice, soups or broths, popsicles, sorbets, ice cubes/chips, nutritional supplements, or sports drinks to help keep you hydrated.

How much water? Calculated by multiplying your weight (in pounds) by 0.67.

Weight (in pounds)	Amount of water per day (in ounces) *
100	67
110	74
120	80
130	87
140	94
150	100
160	107
170	114
180	121
190	127
200	134
210	141
220	148
230	154
240	161
250	168

*More liquids will be required if there is vomiting or diarrhea.

If you are receiving oxaliplatin (Eloxatin) for treatment of pancreatic or colorectal cancer, remember to avoid cold foods or drinks for four to five days after your treatment. Everything that you touch, eat, or drink should be room temperature or warmer.

WHEN NAUSEA AND VOMITING HIT!

1. If the thought or taste of liquid makes you nauseated, give it some time. Slowly sip on non-carbonated (no bubbles), room temperature liquids like water, flat sprite or ginger ale, Gatorade, Powerade, Pedialyte, or other electrolyte replacement drinks. Try diluting your drink (one cup water to one cup clear liquid) to prevent diarrhea from full strength liquids.

2. Start with one teaspoon of a warm temperature, clear liquid every five to ten minutes; increase to one tablespoon every twenty minutes if the liquid is staying down.

3. Remain upright for at least two to three hours after taking in fluids.

4. Try a suppository (absorbed rectally) or orally dissolving nausea medications (examples: Promethazine suppository and Ondansetron orally dissolving tablet).

5. After going four to six hours without vomiting, try bland foods like crackers, rice, toast, dry cereal, soup, or broth.

6. Call your doctor if nausea and/or vomiting last for more than one or two days or if you have the following symptoms: decreased urine output, dark urine, lightheadedness, fever, bloody vomit, bile (yellow or green bitter vomit), headache, or muscle cramps.

7. Ask your doctor if you should continue taking blood pressure medicines, especially diuretics (examples: furosemide, bumetanide, ethacrynic acid, torsemide, hydrochlorothiazide, chlorthalidone, chlorothiazide, metolazone, amiloride, indapamide, spironolactone, triamterene, eplerenone, etc.), while you are nauseated. If your oral intake of liquids and solids is down, your blood pressure may be low, and a blood pressure medicine may not be required. This change may be temporary.

The day of CAT scans/CT scans/computed tomography: In most cases, on the day of CAT scans, there will need to be a four- to six-hour period of fasting. For example, if you have CAT scans at 8:00 a.m., there can be no eating after 2:00 or 4:00 a.m. Your specific institution or hospital will give detailed instructions on when you should have your last meal before scans, or whether you should take your home medications with small sips of water before the exam.

PET Imaging: The day before a PET scan, patients should follow a low-carbohydrate diet—such as non-starchy green vegetables, meat, and eggs—and, like CAT scans, there should be a four- to six-hour period of fasting before the PET scan. Your specific institution or hospital will give detailed instructions on when you should have your last meal before scans and whether you should take your home medications with small sips of water before the exam.

Altered Taste Sensation: Cancer and chemotherapy can alter the taste of both foods and liquids. It is common for patients to note a metallic or bitter taste, often associated with their favorite foods. This can worsen nausea and vomiting and lead to food avoidance. Here are a few tips that patients have offered over the years: Try sucking on a mint or ginger candy to prevent the bitter, metallic taste associated with having your port flushed. Proteins like beef or chicken may not be as enjoyable after chemotherapy; try proteins like fish with fresh lemon or herbs to prevent the metallic taste. Well-washed, fresh fruits and vegetables taste best. Try water with lemon, mint, cucumber, or orange slices.

Honey and Mint Lemonade

Ingredients:

½ cup honey

Juice from 5 lemons

1 cup fresh mint leaves

6 cups cold water

Optional: lemon slices, mint ice cubes (Put a fresh mint leaf in each cell of an ice cube tray with water and freeze until solid)

Instructions:

1. Heat 1 cup of water in a small pot. Stir in honey until it dissolves. Then add fresh mint leaves. Muddle the leaves with a large spoon.

2. Pour the mixture into the remaining 5 cups of cold water.

3. Add lemon juice and stir.

4. Pour and enjoy with lemon slices and/or mint ice cubes!

Cancer Anorexia: One of the most distressing symptoms associated with cancer and chemotherapy is anorexia, or lack of an appetite. The anorexia is not only anxiety-provoking for the patient, it also causes a great deal of anxiety for family members and loved ones. Because of the release of cytokines, cancer patients may have little or no interest in food. All too often, I have seen well-meaning friends and family spend precious time and, in some cases, last days fretting over how little food or drink is being consumed by the cancer patient.

Instead of being preoccupied with food, here are a few suggestions. For the cancer patient undergoing chemotherapy, make small, easy-to-digest meals readily available. Refrain from nagging or haggling over missed meals. In most cases, the cancer patient's appetite will return within days after chemotherapy. Your doctor may suggest medications to help stimulate the appetite, but know that results are mixed. As stated earlier, it is important to maintain adequate fluid hydration when food intake is low.

For the dying patient, cancer anorexia continues to be a major source of anxiety for family and friends. Although it is difficult for us to imagine, however, the dying patient does not have pain or anxiety associated with anorexia. Instead, I suggest that the focus be placed on the comfort of your loved one. She or he may be comforted by a family member's quiet presence, soft music, hearing readings from a favorite book or poem, or by simply having someone to hold their hand.

CHAPTER 5
Cancer and Vaccinations

Talking to patients and their families about vaccinations is tricky. Because there is so much false information out there, and so many misconceptions and myths, often physicians feel as if they are fighting an uphill battle. I happen to think that it is a battle worth fighting, not just for my cancer patients and cancer survivors, but for all patients.

In 2000, when I was a young intern, I witnessed something that had a lasting impression on me as a physician, as a mom, and as a wife. The medical team that I was working with for the day was called to a code blue for a young woman in the medical intensive care unit. A code blue is called in hospitals when a patient loses the ability to breathe on their own or if the heart stops beating. It is the rather dramatic part of medical television dramas, with crash carts and dozens of medical personnel crowded in a room doing chest compressions and sometimes telling everyone to "clear!" as an electric shock is delivered to a dying patient. This scenario was no different. The part of the story that will always stay with me is that this young woman did not survive. Later, as we discussed the case, I was horrified to learn that she died from medical complications of the flu. The way that I looked at this highly preventable illness changed forever.

When it comes to cancer patients on chemotherapy or radiation, survivors of cancer, and their caregivers, I cannot overemphasize the importance of influenza vaccinations every year. The flu season usually starts in October and has a peak number of cases in December and February. In 2018–2019, the CDC reported about 40 million cases of the flu, with 500,000 hospitalizations and approximately 50,000 deaths from complications of the flu. Here is what every cancer patient on chemotherapy, cancer survivor, and cancer caregiver should know about flu vaccinations:

1. Talk to your cancer physician or primary care physician about a flu shot every September or October. The flu shot is a dead virus and cannot give you the flu. On the other hand, the nasal mist that is sometimes offered does have live virus components. It should not be given to cancer patients or their caregivers.

2. Response/immunity to the flu from the vaccine lasts for approximately six months. A flu shot in October will get you through the peak flu months in most cases. If the number of flu cases persists past the spring, talk to your physician about re-vaccination.

3. If you are on chemotherapy, you should get your flu shot two weeks before your next cycle of treatment. This is recommended because it takes about two weeks for the immune system to respond to the vaccination.

4. If you are exposed to the flu, notify your cancer physician or primary care physician about treatment to prevent the flu or to shorten the course of the illness.

Questions about other vaccinations are common from patients receiving chemotherapy and radiation therapy. A simple rule of thumb is this: if it is a live vaccine, it should be avoided. Also, for patients who have undergone a bone marrow transplant, your transplant center and transplant physician will have protocols in place for re-vaccination after transplant. Follow their protocol! Here is a list of recommended vaccines and a schedule for cancer patients and survivors:

Vaccine	Schedule
Influenza (flu) shot	Every year
Tetanus, diphtheria, Pertussis (Tdap)	One Tdap vaccine with a booster every 10 years
Zoster (shingles) *Shingrix only: non-live vaccine*	Two doses between 2 to 6 months apart
Pneumococcal (PCV 13)	One dose
Pneumococcal (PPSV23)	One or two doses
Inactivated Polio shot (4 weeks before chemotherapy or radiation)	One dose if a low antibody level is detected

The need for some vaccines is not clear-cut in cancer patients, and each case should be evaluated individually. The HPV vaccine, for example, can protect against cancers associated with the human papilloma virus, or HPV. HPV is a common and widespread sexually transmitted virus. The vaccine to prevent HPV is most effective when given before sexual exposure to the virus for the prevention of anal, cervical, penile, throat and tonsillar, and vaginal and vulvar cancer. Ideally the vaccine is given around the age of eleven to twelve years old. At the very latest, girls should receive the HPV vaccine by age twenty-six and boys by age twenty-one.

Here is a list of vaccines that should be discussed with your physician:

Vaccine	Schedule
HPV vaccine	3 doses through age 26 (women) or 21 (men)
Meningococcal	Varies
Hepatitis A	Varies
Hepatitis B	Varies

Vaccine	Schedule
Measles, mumps, rubella	Avoid
Influenza nasal mist	Avoid
Zoster (shingles) Zostavix live vaccine	Avoid
Varicella (chicken pox)	Avoid
Smallpox	Avoid
Oral Polio vaccine live virus	Avoid

Live vaccines should be avoided completely in cancer patients, and in some cases (like with the influenza mist) in cancer caregivers.

CHAPTER 6

The Economic Impact of a Cancer Diagnosis

A cancer diagnosis is expensive. According to the National Cancer Institute's Cancer Trends Progress Report from February 2019, cancer care in the United States cost an estimated $137 billion in 2010. Those costs continue to rise, with the price of most new cancer drugs being about $100,000 per patient annually, according to Dr. Barbara K. Rimer of the National Cancer Institute in her March 2018 paper entitled "The Imperative of Addressing Cancer Drug Costs and Value." As a part of new initiatives to involve patients in every aspect of care, treatment planning will include discussing the cost of cancer therapies with the patients, rather than leaving that to insurance companies. Would the high cost of a cancer drug keep you from seeking life-extending or life-saving therapy?

From the cost of chemotherapy drugs, copayments for doctors' visits, and imaging studies, to time lost from work, the economic impact on a patient and his/her family can be devastating. Copayments can vary from nothing to fifty or sixty dollars for a specialist visit. Speak with your doctor about how often you will have a face-to-face visit that requires a copayment, as opposed to an infusion visit that may not require a copayment. Obviously, if there are side effects or issues related to your treatment that require a visit, the cost of the copayment should not be a reason to skip a visit.

Like the doctors' visits, there may be out-of-pocket costs associated with imaging studies, like computed tomography (CT or CAT scans), MRI scans, or PET imaging. Because these studies are so important in the management of cancer, it is necessary to have them done when your doctor orders them. Hospitals may be able to arrange a payment plan or offer the test at a reduced cost if you are unable to afford the copayment. For many cancer patients who have metastatic cancer, those who are undergoing active surveillance, and those on maintenance treatment, CT/CAT scans or PET imaging may be required every three or four months to help guide therapy.

There are numerous charities and foundations available to help with the costs associated with cancer care. Some foundations will cover the out-of-pocket expenses not covered by traditional insurance companies. Others may help with incidentals like transportation, expenses, or meals. To see if the drug company that manufactures your chemotherapy drug has a patient assistance program, check its website.

Some nonprofit programs that help patients with cancer are listed below:

- American Cancer Society—www.cancer.org
- PhRMA's Medicine Assistance Tool (MAT)—www. medicineassistancetool.org

- CancerCare—www.cancercare.org
- CancerCare Co-Payment Assistance Foundation—www.cancercarecopay.org
- Good Days—www.mygooddays.org
- HealthWell Foundation—www.healthwellfoundation.org
- Patient Advocate Foundation's Colorectal Careline—www.colorectalcareline.org
- Patient Advocate Foundation Co-Pay Relief Program—www.copays.org
- Patient Access Network Foundation—www.panfoundation.org
- Patient Services Incorporated—www.patientservicesinc.org
- The Leukemia and Lymphoma Society's Co-Pay Assistance Program—www.lls.org/copay
- Lymphoma Research Foundation—www.lymphoma.org
- United Way—www.unitedway.org

When possible, speak with your human resources office about resources available through your employer. There are programs that donate vacation hours to employees facing critical illnesses that may allow you to receive paid leave. Additionally, speak to your doctor about arranging treatments around your work schedule or on Fridays to allow for weekend recovery time.

Finally, fill out the Family and Medical Leave Act (FMLA) Medical Certification forms and take them to your physician to be completed. FMLA has been in place since 1993 and guarantees certain employees up to twelve weeks of protected leave for qualifying medical conditions. This law also protects the health benefits of the employee.

CHAPTER 7

When Cancer Progresses

Once a patient has been diagnosed with cancer, life is never the same. It is true that cancer patients have a different perspective on life. A longtime patient who is also a minister told me once, "I am on the 50-yard line. Either way it goes, there is victory." Interestingly, he shared this with me at a time when his cancer had relapsed. His diffuse large B-cell lymphoma that had not been detectable for several years had suddenly reappeared without warning. He had been completely symptom free. Though his outlook was optimistic, that is not always the case.

There are patients who put their lives on hold and stop living for fear of a cancer recurrence. Every symptom, no matter how small, is a certain sign of cancer recurrence, and they continually relive the agony of a cancer diagnosis. After over a decade of practice, I have noticed the agony, the "scanxiety," that so many patients feel as they wait for the results of their imaging or surveillance studies. This anxiety is part of the reason why I do not use the words *remission* or *cure* very often. Simply put, they are really confusing and tricky words that convey a certainty about cancer that none of us have.

Remission is still used by doctors to indicate that there is no evidence of cancer seen on CAT scans, PET scans, or blood work. The reason that this word is so complicated, however, is that a cancer recurrence may be so small at first that we are unable to detect it on scans or in bloodwork. Likewise, the word *cure* is confusing. For years, oncologists would tell patients that if they made it to the five-year mark without recurrence, then they were "cured." Today we are much more cautious with the word *cure*, as all of us have seen patients with disease recurrence years or decades out from their initial diagnosis. A wise medical malpractice attorney once told me, "The only thing that you can tell a patient after a CAT scan or PET scan is, 'Yes, you have cancer,' or 'I don't know.'" There is a lot of truth to that statement. Yet we still do CAT scans and PET scans for surveillance in some cases, because for now it is the best that we *can* do.

What is meant by surveillance? It's a study, usually imaging, that is done to look for cancer recurrence. Surveillance is a valid strategy in some cancers, but not in others. From the outset of your diagnosis, you should have a clear idea about whether surveillance studies are necessary and which ones, if any, will be done to detect disease recurrence. The most common surveillance tests for solid tumor cancers, like colorectal, lung, and uterine cancer, are CAT scans and PET scans. If it is indicated, ask how often and for how long these studies will be done.

When cancer recurs or progresses it is devastating, but it is not always a death sentence. A recurrence can mean repeat biopsies, additional surgeries, and more chemotherapy and/or radiation. Disease progression can mean changing chemotherapy drugs to attack the cancer in a different way. There are many important questions that you will want to ask your doctor:

1. For ***disease recurrence***, is a cure still possible?

2. Are there other treatments available, like bone marrow transplant?

3. Is surgery an option? Additional chemotherapy or radiation?

4. For ***disease progression***, how many treatments will be done before repeat studies are performed to check for response?

5. What is the response rate to the next line of therapy?

Maintenance treatment can be offered in some cases of recurrent or metastatic cancer. This can be a difficult concept to explain to patients and family members, but consider this—increasingly, cancer is being treated as a chronic disease. What this means is that for patients with recurrent or metastatic cancer, keeping them on chemotherapy indefinitely is an accepted strategy for long-term disease control. Here is an example:

A patient is treated for Stage 2 adenocarcinoma of the lung with surgery followed by chemotherapy. The cancer recurs one year later, with new disease in the lungs and the liver. It is now metastatic cancer. After twelve weeks of intensive three-drug therapy, scans show shrinkage of the cancer in the lungs and the liver and there is no new disease seen. Maintenance therapy with a less intensive, but still effective, two-drug regimen is started.

The important points to emphasize in the previous case are: 1) The patient still has metastatic disease; there is no "down-staging." 2) The two-drug regimen will continue indefinitely if the cancer stays controlled in the lungs and liver with no evidence of new cancer, and if the two drugs are well tolerated by the patient. 3) This is considered maintenance treatment, and it allows some cancers to be treated as a chronic, long-term disease.

When cure is no longer the goal of therapy, patients and their families will need to tackle some difficult issues. Often, patients and families will avoid these discussions while the cancer patient is doing well, only to raise the issue when there is a crisis. I think that it is easier to discuss the difficult issues while the patient is doing well and able to offer meaningful input. One of the easiest ways to approach difficult topics like end-of-life issues, do-not-resuscitate orders, nutrition, and health care decision making is with a living will. This document makes the patient's wishes known in the event they are unable to speak for themselves.

Start by talking to your doctor. They can help you to understand many of the choices that you will have to make in completing the living will document. Consider these questions:

1. Do you want life support? Under what circumstances would life support or life-sustaining measures like mechanical ventilation, tube feeding/intravenous nutrition, and intravenous fluids be appropriate?

2. Do you want to be resuscitated if your heart stops beating? This would require CPR, or in some cases cardioversion or defibrillation.

3. Who would be your spokesperson? Often, patients will choose a spouse, partner, or child. Make sure that your spokesperson will be guided by facts and not by emotion.

Finally, prepare your document with the help of an attorney or online resources. Your hospital or doctor's office may have a sample document to make preparation easier. Once you have completed the document, be sure to share it with your family and health care providers. A sample living will is attached in the appendix of this book.

In 2014, I was seeing a patient in the hospital who was dying from metastatic lung cancer. Lance* had been to my office multiple times with his wife, Julie*, and his daughter for routine visits. He did well for a while, but after many months of treatment, it became clear that Lance's cancer was progressing. Much to my surprise, as Lance continued to decline, Julie and his daughter made it clear to me that they were not aware of what his end-of-life wishes were. Fortunately, Lance had prepared a living will in my office that outlined his wishes not to be maintained on life support (for example, either mechanical ventilation or tube feeding) and that he did not want to be resuscitated when his heart stopped. Because of the living will, Lance's wife was spared the anguish of having to make difficult decisions when her husband was actively dying.

End-of-life care is a complex and controversial topic for which people have very strong opinions. Ultimately, the conversation always circles back to two topics: quality of life versus quantity of life, and the cost (emotional and financial) of end-of-life care. Is it better to live a shorter amount of time without doctor and hospital visits, or is longevity and more time with one's family the goal? Even as you are reading this book, there are conversations among other medical professionals about the appropriate way to manage end-of-life care. I submit that there is no single, best way. End-of-life care and the journey that each patient takes to get there is as individual as we are. I have patients who opt to stop chemotherapy even when there are other treatment options left. This is the right choice for them. On the other hand, I have patients who choose to go with a third-, fourth-, or fifth-line treatment with the full knowledge that the response rate is extremely low. I believe that this is the right choice for them. What motivates patients and families to make the choices that they make is varied, and can range from financial considerations to absence or presence of a strong social support network to a previous negative experience with the healthcare system.

Recently, I cared for a delightful and spirited sixty-five-year-old woman, Faith*, who had metastatic colorectal cancer. At her initial presentation, Faith's cancer had already spread to the liver. She understood very clearly that she had an incurable disease. After the first line of treatment, Faith had a partial response as expected and went on maintenance treatment. She had a good response to chemotherapy and radiation for nearly two years before her cancer stopped responding to treatment. Our discussions were very open and honest about what her goals were. Her children were mature adults and her husband had recently recovered from a very serious acute illness. She felt that her life's work had been completed, and she decided not to pursue additional palliative (non-curative) chemotherapy even though other treatments were available. For Faith, the next step in her journey did not include chemotherapy; however, it was still important to make sure that quality of life was maintained for Faith and her family. We decided that it was time for hospice.

What is hospice? Hospice is just one form of palliative or supportive care for patients with an incurable illness. Hospice focuses on relieving or preventing suffering related to a cancer diagnosis or other non-curable illnesses. There are studies showing that hospice can improve a patient's length of survival. Hospice improves quality of life as well. It is not the only form of palliative or supportive care. Other palliative or supportive care treatments include chemotherapy, radiation, or other medicines used to manage chronic diseases when a cure is not expected.

This is how I think of palliative care:

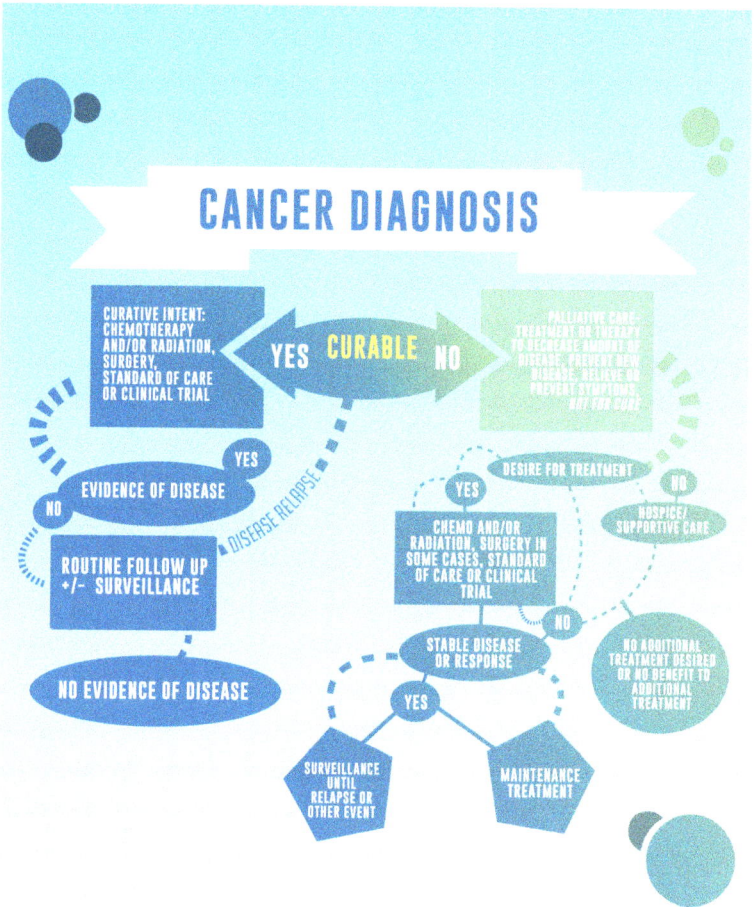

CANCER DIAGNOSIS

CURABLE — YES / NO

CURATIVE INTENT: CHEMOTHERAPY AND/OR RADIATION, SURGERY, STANDARD OF CARE OR CLINICAL TRIAL

PALLIATIVE CARE: TREATMENT OR THERAPY TO DECREASE AMOUNT OF DISEASE, PREVENT NEW DISEASE, RELIEVE OR PREVENT SYMPTOMS. NOT FOR CURE.

EVIDENCE OF DISEASE — YES / NO

DISEASE RELAPSE

ROUTINE FOLLOW UP +/- SURVEILLANCE

NO EVIDENCE OF DISEASE

DESIRE FOR TREATMENT — YES / NO

HOSPICE/ SUPPORTIVE CARE

CHEMO AND/OR RADIATION, SURGERY IN SOME CASES, STANDARD OF CARE OR CLINICAL TRIAL

STABLE DISEASE OR RESPONSE — YES / NO

NO ADDITIONAL TREATMENT DESIRED OR NO BENEFIT TO ADDITIONAL TREATMENT

SURVEILLANCE UNTIL RELAPSE OR OTHER EVENT

MAINTENANCE TREATMENT

To qualify for hospice, a doctor must verify that a patient has an incurable illness with a life expectancy of less than six months. There are often multiple hospice organizations in each city or community, and they will all follow similar guidelines for palliative or supportive care. You, your family, and your doctor should work together to decide when hospice care is appropriate. Will every cancer patient with an incurable disease go on hospice? No. In some cases, cancer patients will die from complications unrelated to their cancer diagnosis. In other cases, patients may choose to continue aggressive therapy until late in the disease process. Some call this futile care; however, because each case is different, I encourage families and other medical providers to withhold judgment of the dying patient.

An example of a patient who did not pursue hospice immediately was Tracy*. Tracy was in her late thirties when she presented with metastatic, or Stage 4, triple negative breast cancer in January 2018. She had a large breast mass along with brain, lung, liver, and bone metastases noted at the initial visit. Tracy's only request at our first visit was to see her daughter graduate from high school. There was a good response to first-line treatment; however, it was not long before new areas of disease were noted in the lungs and liver. Tracy went through multiple rounds of chemotherapy and radiation for her breast cancer, all with a mixed response. There were some areas of improvement, but other areas showed continued progression of the breast cancer. In July 2019, Tracy and I had a lengthy discussion about the risks versus benefits of continuing with chemotherapy. After multiple rounds of treatment, it seemed unlikely that we would see a meaningful response from additional lines of therapy. Tracy had one last request, however. She wanted to be able to visit with her mother, who lived in another state, for a final time. We were able to honor her wish, and when she was ready to go on hospice, the appropriate referrals were made. Did Tracy's journey look like anyone else's journey? It did not. Did she live out her days on her own terms? She did.

CHAPTER 8

Understanding Clinical Trials

Clinical trials have a long, troubling, and complicated history. For many in the United States, especially African Americans from the South, the mention of clinical trials conjures up images of Alabama and the Tuskegee Syphilis Study. This study recorded the natural history of 600 African American men: 399 with syphilis and 201 without syphilis. The study went on for forty years. The 600 men never gave informed consent to be observed. Sadly, even when penicillin became widely recognized as the treatment of choice for syphilis in 1945, the remaining survivors with syphilis were never offered treatment, as the scientists involved wished to study the end stages of the disease. Instead, they were offered free medical exams, free meals, and burial insurance. A multi-million-dollar court settlement in 1974 attempted to compensate for the harms done in the Tuskegee Syphilis Study. The settlement provided health and medical benefits to survivors, and eventually to their offspring.

Today, clinical trials are strictly regulated by review boards. Trials are carefully designed to ensure that patient volunteers are not harmed. Patients in clinical trials receive a study-drug, a placebo (no active treatment or a "sugar pill"), or the standard of care medicines (the usual treatment), as well as blood tests, imaging studies, exams, and doctor's visits at no cost to them while they are enrolled on the study. Depending on the design of the study, patients may be randomly assigned (luck of the draw) to a treatment arm in a blinded fashion. Blinded means that the patient and physician are unaware of which treatment the patient is receiving. This prevents bias when looking at outcomes in a clinical trial. Patients are required to give informed consent, but they are also given the opportunity to withdraw from a clinical trial at any time without being penalized.

In cancer medicine, clinical trials have helped to obtain Food and Drug Administration (FDA) approval for numerous life-extending and life-saving drugs. In order to be approved by the FDA, new cancer drugs, like other drugs on the market, must demonstrate a benefit in clinical trials over older treatments or no treatment. In some cases, clinical trials have also shown the benefit of adding new drugs to an existing regimen.

There are multiple important phases to a clinical trial. A phase I trial asks whether an experimental drug or therapy is **safe.** A phase II study asks whether the experimental therapy is **effective.** A phase III study asks if the experimental therapy **works better than an existing approved therapy**. If the answer is yes, the drug is submitted to the FDA to be an approved therapy. A phase IV study takes already approved therapies and evaluates **safety over time.**

There are circumstances in cancer medicine when considering a clinical trial is especially appealing: 1) For treatment of rare cancers that do not have effective and established therapies. 2) For patients who have been through and exhausted multiple lines of established treatments and their cancer is no longer responding. 3) When there is an option to add an experimental therapeutic agent to an already established and effective regimen in hopes of improving the response rate.

Patients on clinical trials are monitored very closely for expected and unexpected side effects from the study drug(s). Additionally, because of the interest in the new agent's effectiveness, imaging with CAT scans or PET scans may be requested more frequently. For imaging that is required more frequently than the accepted guidelines, the costs of these tests will generally be covered by the investigator.

Clinical trials for new cancer therapies may be offered by your medical or radiation oncologist. For more information about clinical trials in the United States and abroad, go to www.clinicaltrials.gov.

CHAPTER 9
Surviving the Long-Term Side Effects

Getting through chemotherapy is not the end of a cancer survivor's journey. Many patients deal with long-term side effects of treatments for years, and in some cases for the rest of their lives. While there may be medications available to help with particular side effects, some of these treatments are only minimally effective. In some cases, encouraging patients to accept a new normal after chemotherapy is important to help them move forward in their journey.

There are some non-drug-related strategies that may be helpful. Exercise may be a useful therapy to help combat debilitating fatigue. With exercise, the body releases natural mood-lifting hormones called endorphins. With thirty to forty-five minutes of exercise at least four or five days weekly, not only do cancer survivors experience less fatigue and feel better generally, but exercise may also lower the risk of cancer recurrence.

Debilitating fatigue may also be a consequence of poor sleep hygiene. Rejuvenating, restorative sleep is best achieved in a room cooled to 70 degrees Fahrenheit with no light or noise. All devices, including televisions, radios, cellular phones, and tablets, should be silenced or powered off. A consistent bedtime and wake time, even on the weekends and holidays, will promote more effective and restful sleep.

There are other important long-term side effects of cancer therapy that are important to discuss with your doctor. Ask your physician if your previous cancer treatment puts you at increased risk for secondary cancers, thyroid dysfunction, or early heart disease. Also, make sure that appropriate screening tests and blood studies are being performed at the correct age. Inquire about whether your chemotherapy, especially if given at a young age, will affect your ability to have children. Certain surgeries, for example orchiectomy (having the testicles surgically removed) for young males with testicular cancer, will prevent them from being able to father children. Likewise, chemotherapy can lead to premature menopause or ovarian dysfunction in some women.

Over the years, I have treated several young patients for Hodgkin's lymphoma. Hodgkin's lymphoma has extremely high cure rates, and as such, the approach, particularly because the patients are young, is aggressive. The youngest patient that I have ever treated, Teresa*, presented with a large mass in her chest that compressed her heart and lungs. Although she responded very well to standard chemotherapy, radiation therapy to the remaining disease in the chest was required to increase the chance of cure. With that additional therapy comes the increased risk of secondary cancer, specifically breast cancer. Additionally, Teresa will be at increased risk for an inactive or underactive thyroid as well as early heart disease due to radiation therapy. She will require ongoing oncology follow-up, early screening mammography, thyroid function studies, and close follow-up with cardiology (a physician trained in diseases of the heart) for the rest of her life. The goal of therapy is cure, but sometimes it comes with a price.

CHAPTER 10

Reducing Cancer Risk

The risk of developing cancer is influenced by several factors. Some of these factors, called non-modifiable risk factors, are beyond our control. Examples include genetics, family history, gender, and age. It is known that certain ethnic groups have an increased risk for certain cancers. Women of Ashkenazi Jewish ancestry, for example, have a one in forty risk of carrying a BRCA1 or BRCA2 mutation. This increases the risk of developing breast and ovarian cancer. With this knowledge, recommendations should be made for risk-reducing surgery, with prophylactic (before a cancer develops) bilateral mastectomy (removal of both breasts) and removal of both ovaries once childbearing is completed. Additionally, family history, gender, and increasing age can increase the risk for certain cancers. Breast cancer is far more common in women than men. Likewise, older women have a higher risk for breast cancer than younger women. There are no proven risk-reduction strategies for gender and age.

Modifiable risk factors are the risk factors that we can control. Some of these modifiable risk factors include diet, social habits like smoking or alcohol use, and weight. Diet and weight are closely linked. There is indisputable data linking being overweight and obesity to multiple health-related problems, including cancer, heart disease, and stroke. Because of the connection between fat cells and estrogen production, it is known that obesity is a risk factor not only for developing breast cancer, but for recurrence of cancer in breast cancer survivors as well. The body mass index, or BMI, is calculated using your weight and height (weight in kilograms divided by the height in meters squared). See nhlbi.nih.gov for a BMI calculator. A BMI between 18.5 and 24.9 indicates that you are a healthy weight for your height. A BMI of 25–29.9 indicates that you are overweight. A BMI of 30 or higher indicates that you are obese.

Smoking has been linked to an increased risk of nearly every cancer. Though it is common to think of lung cancer and tobacco use, it is well known that smokers are at increased risk of pancreatic, kidney, bladder, esophageal, and head and neck cancers. Never smoking is the most effective strategy to prevent tobacco-associated cancers. Although the risk for smoking-related cancers goes down when one stops smoking, a former smoker's risk of certain cancers is never as low as the nonsmoker's risk. Stopping smoking is important for reducing cancer recurrence. Additionally, not smoking improves a cancer patient's response to chemotherapy.

The data on alcohol and cancer risk and recurrence is less clear. What is clear is that drinking in excessive amounts increases the risk of developing breast, colorectal, esophageal, pancreatic, and head and neck cancer. Excessive amounts of alcohol can increase the risk of recurrence of these same cancers. According to federal guidelines, heavy drinking is defined as four or more alcoholic beverages on any day or more than eight per week for women, and five or more alcoholic beverages on any day or more than fifteen per week for men.

When patients ask what they can do to lower their risk of developing cancer, or to lower their risk of cancer recurrence, the answer is simple:

1. Refrain from excessive amounts of alcohol use.
2. Eat a well-balanced and healthy diet with little or no processed foods.
3. Maintain a healthy weight.
4. Exercise regularly (three or four times weekly for thirty to forty-five minutes).
5. Refrain from smoking.
6. Get adequate amounts of rest.

Of course, there are no guarantees. Many of the patients that I care for with advanced malignancy have no family history of cancer, have never smoked and are non-drinkers, and maintain healthy, active lifestyles. Life is tricky!

CHAPTER 11

Being a Survivor—Faith, Not Fear

Survivorship starts at the moment that a cancer diagnosis is made and continues for a lifetime. Initially, all the focus is on outlining the most effective treatment strategies and minimizing treatment-related toxicities. At the conclusion of treatment, however, survivorship is about managing life with a new normal—either as a cancer-free survivor or as one living with cancer.

Often, there is so much emphasis on the cancer diagnosis that patients and providers may forget about chronic illnesses. It is always tragic when patients complete their cancer treatment only to suffer or die from complications of another chronic illness, like diabetes, hypertension, heart disease, or stroke. It is vitally important to continue to follow up with primary care doctors and to continue taking medications as previously prescribed. This is important for both the cancer-free survivor and those living with cancer.

I have images of two survivors that I would like to share. Both are breast cancer survivors. One lives daily with cancer and the other lives as a cancer-free survivor.

The first patient, Rose*, presented with metastatic breast cancer in 2017. She had disease in her lungs and liver, but was functioning quite well. Rose had a wonderful support network and worked at a job that she enjoyed every day. On our very first visit, I changed the entire treatment plan that the surgeon had laid out, and in doing so I was certain that I had lost her confidence. When I explained that her metastatic cancer would not benefit from surgery and was treatable but not curable, Rose and her family were visibly shaken. Days later, with her family by her side, Rose quickly rallied her confidence and came back to my office to start chemotherapy. She has done well for nearly two years, and continues to work at the same job that she enjoys. Some of our best conversations have centered around what it means to her to be a cancer survivor. She is not sad for herself. She does not start conversations with, "I am a cancer survivor." In fact, many people are unaware of her breast cancer or that she has been on chemotherapy continuously for the past two years. Although Rose's cancer is not curable, she has not given up on life, and her journey with cancer is still being written.

The second patient, Christine*, was diagnosed with bilateral triple negative breast cancer in 2013. Triple negative breast cancer is more commonly seen in African American and Hispanic women, and is more aggressive, has no targets to treat, and has a higher risk for recurrence. After undergoing bilateral mastectomy, Christine completed six difficult months of chemotherapy. She had a very supportive group of family and friends who were constantly by her side. At the completion of her treatment, I proudly entered the room and excitedly announced that at last she had gotten through chemotherapy. Her journey was complete. She gazed at me with a puzzled look, and said, "What am I supposed to do now? What will I do every week without chemotherapy treatments?" I, too, was puzzled. It was one of the first times that a patient had communicated so clearly the anxiety she felt when there was no more active treatment to take. What I considered a milestone in completing a hard task was for Christine the beginning of watching and waiting for some terrible recurrence of her cancer. My mistake was in thinking that Christine's journey was complete. In fact, her journey was just beginning. We have spent the past six years quietly reassuring her that her cancer does not have to come back. Every visit gets a little easier as I watch Christine focus more on the victories that she has experienced over the past six years, rather than the defeats. She has watched grandchildren grow, a daughter has overcome personal challenges, and she has managed to find joy in working out and dating again. Does it mean that her cancer will never come back? It does not. But finding joy again after a cancer diagnosis does mean that cancer is not winning.

One of my most inspiring patients was a local celebrity and hero to many. He liked to say that we were both winners. He won on the basketball court and I won in the chemotherapy suite. I did not know Lewis* before his metastatic lung cancer diagnosis, but my frequent conversations with him at his doctor's visits quickly made him more than a patient. He was my friend. Lewis lived by the phrase "Faith, not fear!" He gave out black bracelets with this phrase imprinted boldly in white, and I saw firsthand how it inspired others who were trying to survive as well. When he spoke with others about his incurable cancer, his message was clear: Lewis did not fear cancer and he did not fear dying. Lewis lived well and had many successes, all while taking chemotherapy. When he died, we were all deeply saddened, but we were also grateful. I remain grateful that I had the chance to witness a journey that focused on the fullness of life. A journey that focused on faith, not fear.

CHAPTER 12

What I Have Learned

I have learned a lot in my twelve years as a cancer physician, and I am sure that I will learn more. Over the years, I have frequently told my patients that I gain so much more from them than I could ever give back. My patients have ranged from preachers to pimps (it's true), and ninety-year-olds to nineteen-year-olds. There has been a fair of amount time spent just talking about lives lived and regrets over things that will be missed. As emotionally exhausting as it can be, talking about cancer all day, every day, I really cannot imagine doing anything else. Even in the tough seasons, when patients' cancers progress or someone dies unexpectedly, I know that my staff and I will be rejuvenated by the successes that come our way.

What I have learned is that we can only be defeated by that of which we are afraid. My patients have taught me to live each day to the fullest and to approach life and death with courage. If you have ever been with a family member or friend when they are actively dying (an oxymoron, right?), it is a shocking reminder of the differences between life and death. A birth is filled with chaos and noise—think labor and delivery nurses, a crying newborn, and perhaps a fainting father. Death, on the other hand, when it is done with dignity, is a peaceful and calm transition. Thankfully, not all my patients die from cancer or cancer-related complications. But for those patients whose lives will be shortened by cancer, I pray that they will have a peaceful transition, and I pray for comfort for those of us left behind.

"I have told you these things, so that in me you may have peace. In this world you will have trouble. But take heart! I have overcome the world." John 16:33 (NIV)

Thank You

I am so grateful for the hundreds of patients and families who I have had the opportunity to know and care for, since I started my career in cancer medicine as a subspecialty fellow in 2003 at the University of Alabama in Birmingham, up to the present time in private practice at Alabama Oncology Princeton, and briefly at Cooper Green Mercy Hospital. Though the journey has been filled with sad and unpredictable moments, there have been great moments of joy and triumph as well. All through the journey, I have wanted to share some of the things that I have learned along the way. My hope is that some of the tricks of the trade will make the reader's cancer journey a little easier. Maybe you will remember that life, even when cancer is involved, is all about faith and not fear. I hope that no matter what life has in store for us, we'll always remember that God's grace is enough to get us through. Many thanks to Al, Ryan, and Olivia, who encouraged me to pursue new challenges and move out of my comfort zone.

"Do not be anxious about anything, but in every situation, by prayer and petition, with thanksgiving, present your requests to God." Philippians 4:6 (NIV)

"Now faith is confidence in what we hope for and assurance about what we do not see." Hebrews 11:1 (NIV)

References

Crooks, V, Waller S, et al. The use of the Karnofsky Performance Scale in determining outcomes and risk in geriatric outpatients. J Gerontol. 1991; 46: M139-M144.

de Haan R, Aaronson A, et al. Measuring quality of life in stroke. Stroke. 1993; 24:320- 327.

Hollen PJ, Gralla RJ, et al. Measurement of quality of life in patients with lung cancer in multicenter trials of new therapies. Cancer. 1994; 73: 2087-2098.

Oken, M.M., Creech, R.H., Tormey, D.C., Horten, J., Davis, T.E., McFadden, E.T., Carbone, P.P, Toxicity and Response Criteria of the Eastern Cooperative Oncology Group. Am J Clin Oncol 5: 649-655, 1982.

O'Toole DM, Golden AM. Evaluating cancer patients for rehabilitation potential. West J Med. 1991; 155:384-387.

Oxford Textbook of Palliative Medicine, Oxford University Press. 1993;109.

Schag CC, Heinrich RL, Ganz PA. Karnofsky performance status revisited: Reliability, validity, and guidelines. J Clin Oncology. 1984; 2:187-193

Appendix

ADVANCE DIRECTIVE FOR HEALTH CARE
(Living Will and Health Care Proxy)

This form may be used to make your wishes known about what medical treatment or other care you would or would not want if you become too sick to speak for yourself. You are not required to have an advance directive. **If you do have an advance directive, be sure that your doctor, family, and friends know you have one and know where it is located.**

Section 1: Living will.

I, _____, being of sound mind and at least 19 years old, would like to make the following wishes known. I direct that my family, my doctors and health care workers, and all others follow the directions I am writing down. I know that at any time I can change my mind about these directions by tearing up this form and writing a new one. I can also do away with these directions by tearing them up and by telling someone at least 19 years of age of my wishes and asking him or her to write them down.

I understand that these directions will only be used if I am not able to speak for myself.

If I become terminally ill or injured:

Terminally ill or injured is when my doctor and another doctor decide that I have a condition that cannot be cured and that I will likely die soon from this condition.

Life-sustaining treatment—Life-sustaining treatment includes drugs, machines, or medical procedures that would keep me alive but would not cure me. I know that even if I choose not to have life-sustaining treatment, I will still get medicines and treatments that ease my pain and keep me comfortable.

Place your initials by either "yes" or "no":

I want to have life-sustaining treatment if I am terminally ill or injured.

_____ Yes   _____ No

Artificially provided food and hydration (Food and water through a tube or an IV)—I understand that if I am terminally ill or injured I may need to be given food and water through a tube or an IV to keep me alive if I can no longer chew or swallow on my own or with someone helping me.

Place your initials by either "yes" or "no":

I want to have food and water provided through a tube or an IV if I am terminally ill or injured.

_____ Yes   _____ No

If I become permanently unconscious:

Permanent unconsciousness is when my doctor and another doctor agree that within a reasonable degree of medical certainty I can no longer think, feel anything, knowingly move, or be aware of being alive. They believe this condition will last indefinitely without hope for improvement and have watched me long enough to make that decision. I understand that at least one of these doctors must be qualified to make such a diagnosis.

Life-sustaining treatment—Life-sustaining treatment includes drugs, machines, or other medical procedures that would keep me alive but would not cure me. I know that even if I choose not to have life-sustaining treatment, I will still get medicines and treatments that ease my pain and keep me comfortable.

Place your initials by either "yes" or "no":

I want to have life-sustaining treatment if I am permanently unconscious.

_____ Yes   _____ No

Artificially provided food and hydration (Food and water through a tube or an IV)—I understand that if I become permanently unconscious, I may need to be given food and water through a tube or an IV to keep me alive if I can no longer chew or swallow on my own or with someone helping me.

Place your initials by either "yes" or "no":

I want to have food and water provided through a tube or an IV if I am permanently unconscious.

_____ Yes   _____ No

Other Directions: Please list any other things you want done or not done.

In addition to the directions I have listed on this form, I also want the following:

_____

_____

_____

_____

If you do not have other directions, place your initials here:

_____ No, I do not have any other directions.

Section 2: If I need someone to speak for me.

This form can be used in the State of Alabama to name a person you would like to have make medical or other decisions for you if you become too sick to speak for yourself. This person is called a healthcare proxy. You do not have to name a healthcare proxy. The directions in this form will be followed even if you do not name a healthcare proxy.

Place your initials by only one answer:

_____ I do not want to name a healthcare proxy. (If you check this answer, go to Section 3.)

_____ I do want the person listed below to be my health care proxy. I have talked with this person about my wishes.

First choice for proxy: _____

Relationship to me: _____

Address: _____

City: _____ State: ____ Zip: _____

Day-time phone number: _____

Night-time phone number: _____

If this person is not able, not willing, or not available to be my health care proxy, this is my next choice:

Second choice for proxy: _____

Relationship to me: _____

Address: _____

City: _____ State: ____ Zip: _____

Day-time phone number: _____

Night-time phone number: _____

Instructions for Proxy:

Place your initials by either "yes" or "no":

I want my health care proxy to make decisions about whether to give me food and water through a tube or an IV.

_____ Yes _____ No

Place your initials by only one of the following:

_____ I want my health care proxy to follow only the directions as listed on this form.

_____ I want my health care proxy to follow my directions as listed on this form and to make any decisions about things I have not covered in the form.

_____ I want my health care proxy to make the final decision, even though it could mean doing something different from what I have listed on this form.

Section 3: The things listed on this form are what I want.

I understand the following:

- If my doctor or hospital does not want to follow the directions I have listed, they must see that I get to a doctor or hospital who will follow my directions.

- If I am pregnant, or if I become pregnant, the choices I have made on this form will not be followed until after the birth of the baby.

- If the time comes for me to stop receiving life sustaining treatment or food and water through a tube or an IV, I direct that my doctor talk about the good and bad points of doing this, along with my wishes, with my health care proxy, if I have one, and with the following people:

_____

_____

Section 4: My signature.

Your name: _____

The month, day, and year of your birth:

_____

Your signature: _____

Date signed: _____

Section 5: Witnesses (need two witnesses to sign)

I am witnessing this form because I believe this person to be of sound mind. I did not sign the person's signature, and I am not the health care proxy. I am not related to the person by blood, adoption, or marriage, and am not entitled to any part of his or her estate. I am at least 19 years of age and am not directly responsible for paying for his or her medical care.

Name of first witness: _____

Signature: _____

Date: _____

Name of first witness: _____

Signature: _____

Date: _____

Section 6: Signature of proxy

I, _____, am willing to serve as the health care proxy.

Signature: _____Date: _____

Signature of second choice for proxy:

I, _____, am willing to serve as the health care proxy if the first choice cannot serve.

Signature: _____Date: _____

Notes

Notes

Notes

Notes

Notes

Notes

Notes

Notes

About the Author

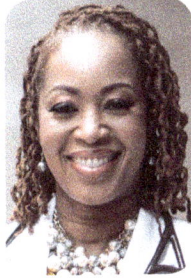

Dr. Katisha Vance is a triple board-certified internist, hematologist, and medical oncologist, as well as an author, speaker, and consultant. She is passionate about helping patients and their families navigate an often confusing, complex, and ever-changing cancer journey, and strives to provide simple, real-world solutions that help patients and their loved ones cope with the physical and emotional challenges of a new cancer diagnosis.

Dr. Katisha earned her MD from the University of Alabama and served as one of three chief medical residents for her internal medicine training program. She is the first college graduate in her family. In her free time, Dr. Katisha is an avid reader and loves gardening. She lives in Birmingham, Alabama, with her husband, Aldos, and their two children, Ryan and Olivia.

Learn more at www.drkatisha.com

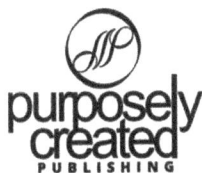

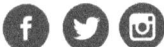

www.ingramcontent.com/pod-product-compliance
Lightning Source LLC
Chambersburg PA
CBHW040756220326
41597CB00029BB/4954